Substantia nigra

Racked by Zeeshan Mahmud

Disclaimer: This book is not authored by a medical doctor or healthcare professional. The information provided within these pages is based on personal research, experiences, and observations, and should not be considered a substitute for professional medical advice, diagnosis, or treatment. It is essential to consult with qualified healthcare professionals for individualized medical guidance and care tailored to your specific needs and circumstances. The author of this book does not assume responsibility for any consequences arising from the use or interpretation of the information presented herein. Readers are encouraged to seek appropriate medical advice and assistance from licensed healthcare providers for any health-related concerns or conditions.

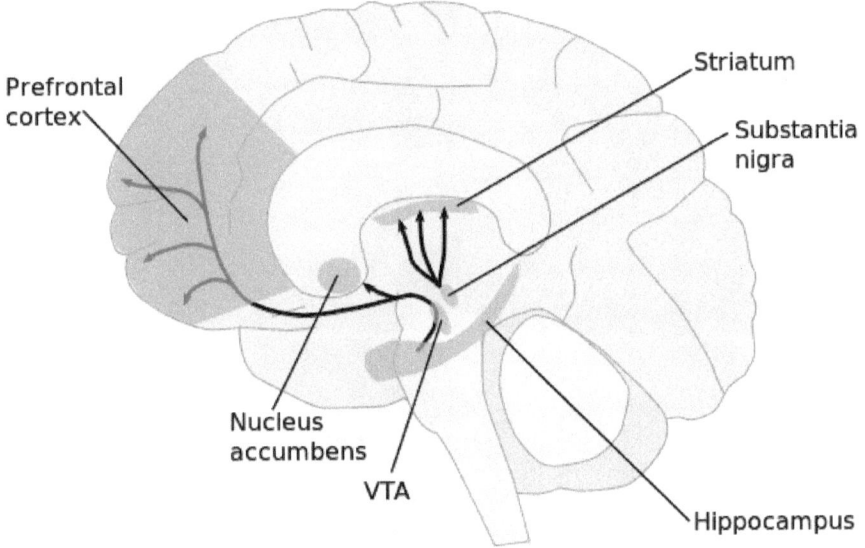

The skinny...

Substantia nigra, or "black substance" in Latin, is a vital component of the brain's basal ganglia, located in the midbrain. It's named for its dark pigmentation, which comes from the presence of neuromelanin, a pigment associated with dopamine-containing neurons. Here's a breakdown:

1. Location and Anatomy: Substantia nigra is found in the midbrain, specifically within the mesencephalon, which is part of the brainstem. It consists of two parts: the pars compacta (SNc) and the pars reticulata (SNr). The SNc contains densely packed dopamine-producing neurons, while the SNr contains mainly GABAergic neurons.

2. Function: The substantia nigra plays a crucial role in movement control and coordination. Its main function is to regulate the initiation and inhibition of voluntary movements. Dopamine, produced by neurons in the SNc, is a neurotransmitter that modulates motor functions, reward, and motivation.

3. Connection with Basal Ganglia: Substantia nigra forms connections with other parts of the basal ganglia, including the striatum (caudate nucleus and putamen) and the globus pallidus. These connections

form the basal ganglia circuit, which is involved in motor control and cognitive functions.

4. Role in Parkinson's Disease: Parkinson's disease is characterized by the degeneration of dopamine-producing neurons in the substantia nigra. This degeneration leads to a reduction in dopamine levels, resulting in the motor symptoms associated with Parkinson's, such as tremors, rigidity, and bradykinesia (slowness of movement).

5. Research and Clinical Significance: Understanding the function and dysfunction of the substantia nigra is crucial for developing treatments for Parkinson's disease and other movement disorders. Researchers are exploring various approaches, including medication, deep brain stimulation, and gene therapy, to alleviate symptoms by targeting the substantia nigra and its connections.

In summary, the substantia nigra is a key brain structure involved in motor control and coordination, primarily through its production of dopamine. Its dysfunction is central to the development of Parkinson's disease, making it a significant area of study in neuroscience and neurology.

Origin story...

Every brain organ has an origin story right? The substantia nigra's origin and discovery are fascinating parts of its history in neuroscience:

1. Origin of Name: The term "substantia nigra" originates from Latin, where "substantia" means substance or matter, and "nigra" means black or dark. This name reflects the structure's distinctive dark coloration due to the presence of neuromelanin pigment.

2. Discovery: The substantia nigra was first described by Félix Vicq-d'Azyr, a French anatomist, in the late 18th century. However, it was not until the 19th century that its significance began to be understood.

3. Early Observations: In the early 19th century, researchers like Moritz Heinrich Romberg and Karl Friedrich Burdach noted the relationship between the substantia nigra and motor function, though their understanding was limited.

4. Key Discoveries: The substantia nigra's importance in movement control was highlighted by Jean-Martin Charcot, a prominent French neurologist, in the mid-19th century. Charcot observed changes in the

substantia nigra in patients with Parkinson's disease, though he mistakenly attributed the condition to changes in the cerebral cortex rather than the midbrain.

5. Later Research: Further advancements in the understanding of the substantia nigra came in the 20th century with the advent of techniques such as histology, neuroimaging, and electrophysiology. Researchers like Arvid Carlsson, who discovered dopamine's role as a neurotransmitter, and Oleh Hornykiewicz, who demonstrated dopamine deficiency in Parkinson's disease, greatly contributed to our understanding of the substantia nigra's function and its involvement in Parkinson's disease.

6. Modern Research: Today, ongoing research continues to elucidate the intricacies of the substantia nigra, its role in motor control, and its implications in neurological disorders such as Parkinson's disease. Advanced imaging techniques, genetic studies, and molecular biology approaches contribute to our evolving understanding of this vital brain structure.

Some history please...

The history of the substantia nigra's discovery and research is a fascinating journey that spans centuries and involves the contributions of many scientists. Here's a brief overview:

1. Early Observations:
   - The term "substantia nigra," which means "black substance" in Latin, was first used by the anatomist Félix Vicq d'Azyr in the late 18th century to describe the darkly pigmented region of the midbrain.
   - Early anatomists noted the presence of this pigmented area but were unsure of its function.

2. Nigrostriatal Pathway:
   - In the late 19th and early 20th centuries, researchers such as Edinger, Meynert, and others began to investigate the connections between different brain regions.
   - They identified a pathway connecting the substantia nigra to the striatum, which would later be known as the nigrostriatal pathway.
   - These early studies laid the groundwork for understanding the role of the substantia nigra in motor control.

3. Dopaminergic Neurons:

- In the mid-20th century, researchers including Arvid Carlsson, Oleh Hornykiewicz, and others made groundbreaking discoveries about the neurotransmitter dopamine and its role in the brain.
   - They identified dopamine as the primary neurotransmitter produced by neurons in the substantia nigra and demonstrated its involvement in motor function.
   - Carlsson and Hornykiewicz's work laid the foundation for understanding dopamine's role in Parkinson's disease and the development of dopamine-based therapies.

4. Parkinson's Disease:
   - The substantia nigra gained significant attention in the study of Parkinson's disease, a neurodegenerative disorder characterized by the degeneration of dopaminergic neurons in this brain region.
   - James Parkinson, a British physician, provided the first detailed description of the disease in his 1817 publication, "An Essay on the Shaking Palsy."
   - Subsequent research, including studies by William Gowers, Jean-Martin Charcot, and others, further elucidated the clinical features and pathology of Parkinson's disease.

5. Modern Research:

- Advances in neuroscience techniques, including neuroimaging, electrophysiology, and molecular biology, have enabled researchers to study the substantia nigra with greater precision.

- Contemporary scientists continue to investigate the role of the substantia nigra in movement, cognition, and disease, as well as potential therapeutic strategies for conditions such as Parkinson's disease.

- Researchers such as Stanley Fahn, Roger Barker, and others have made significant contributions to our understanding of Parkinson's disease and the substantia nigra's involvement.

... & Timeline

1. Discovery by Félix Vicq-d'Azyr (1784):
   - The substantia nigra was first identified by the French anatomist Félix Vicq-d'Azyr in 1784.
   - Vicq-d'Azyr described this structure as a "black substance" due to its dark pigmentation, which distinguished it from surrounding brain tissue.
   - His discovery laid the foundation for subsequent research into the anatomical and functional significance of the substantia nigra.

2. Allusion by Samuel Thomas von Sömmerring (1791):
   - In 1791, the German anatomist Samuel Thomas von Sömmerring made reference to the substantia nigra in his work.
   - Von Sömmerring's acknowledgment of this brain structure further contributed to its recognition within the scientific community.

3. Differentiation by Sano (1910):
   - In 1910, a Japanese neuroanatomist named Sano proposed the differentiation between two main parts of the substantia nigra: the pars reticulata and the pars compacta.

- This distinction highlighted the structural complexity of the substantia nigra and paved the way for more detailed anatomical studies.

4. Hornykiewicz's Contribution (1963):
   - In 1963, Oleh Hornykiewicz, an Austrian pharmacologist, made a significant observation regarding the substantia nigra in Parkinson's disease.
   - Hornykiewicz concluded that the cell loss observed in the substantia nigra of Parkinson's disease patients could be responsible for the dopamine deficit observed in the striatum, a key brain region involved in motor control.
   - This finding provided critical insight into the underlying pathology of Parkinson's disease and laid the groundwork for dopamine-based therapies aimed at restoring neurotransmitter levels in the brain.

These key milestones in the history of the substantia nigra reflect the gradual unraveling of its anatomical, functional, and pathological significance over time. From its initial discovery to contemporary research, scientists have made significant strides in understanding the role of the substantia nigra in health and disease.

Damage to substantia nigra

When there is missing or reduced activity in the substantia nigra, it can lead to significant neurological consequences, particularly in movement control and coordination. Here's what happens:

1. Parkinson's Disease: The most well-known condition associated with dysfunction of the substantia nigra is Parkinson's disease. In Parkinson's, there is a progressive loss of dopamine-producing neurons in the substantia nigra pars compacta (SNc). This loss of neurons leads to a significant reduction in dopamine levels in the brain. Dopamine is essential for regulating movement and coordination. Consequently, the hallmark symptoms of Parkinson's disease include tremors, rigidity, bradykinesia (slowness of movement), and postural instability.

2. Motor Impairments: Reduced dopamine levels due to substantia nigra dysfunction can result in various motor impairments beyond those seen in Parkinson's disease. These may include difficulties with initiating and executing voluntary movements, muscle stiffness, involuntary muscle contractions (dystonia), and impaired balance and gait.

3. Non-Motor Symptoms: Dysfunction in the substantia nigra can also contribute to non-motor symptoms, such as cognitive impairment, mood disturbances (including depression and anxiety), sleep disturbances, autonomic dysfunction (such as constipation and urinary problems), and sensory changes.

4. Other Movement Disorders: While Parkinson's disease is the most common disorder associated with substantia nigra dysfunction, other movement disorders can also result from abnormalities in this brain region. These may include multiple system atrophy (MSA), progressive supranuclear palsy (PSP), and corticobasal degeneration (CBD), among others.

5. Treatment Implications: Understanding the role of the substantia nigra in movement control has led to the development of treatments aimed at restoring dopamine levels in the brain. Medications such as levodopa, dopamine agonists, and MAO-B inhibitors are commonly used to alleviate symptoms of Parkinson's disease by increasing dopamine activity. Deep brain stimulation (DBS) surgery, which involves implanting electrodes into specific brain regions including the substantia nigra, can also help manage symptoms in some cases.

Cause of damage

Damage to the substantia nigra can occur due to various factors, including:

1. Neurodegenerative Diseases: Parkinson's disease is the most common neurodegenerative disorder associated with damage to the substantia nigra. In Parkinson's, there is a progressive loss of dopamine-producing neurons in the substantia nigra pars compacta (SNc). Other neurodegenerative diseases, such as multiple system atrophy (MSA), progressive supranuclear palsy (PSP), and corticobasal degeneration (CBD), can also lead to damage in this brain region.

2. Genetic Factors: Some genetic mutations have been linked to an increased risk of developing Parkinson's disease and other neurodegenerative disorders that affect the substantia nigra. These mutations can disrupt cellular processes involved in maintaining the health and function of neurons in this brain region.

3. Environmental Toxins: Exposure to certain environmental toxins has been implicated in causing damage to the substantia nigra and increasing the risk of developing Parkinson's disease. One

well-known toxin is MPTP (1-methyl-4-phenyl-1,2,3,6-tetrahydropyridine), which can selectively destroy dopamine-producing neurons in the substantia nigra, leading to Parkinsonian symptoms.

4. Oxidative Stress: Oxidative stress, resulting from an imbalance between the production of reactive oxygen species (ROS) and the body's antioxidant defenses, can damage cells in the substantia nigra. This oxidative damage is thought to contribute to the progression of neurodegenerative diseases like Parkinson's.

5. Inflammation: Chronic inflammation in the brain can also contribute to damage in the substantia nigra. Inflammatory processes can activate microglia, the brain's immune cells, leading to neuronal damage and dysfunction. Inflammatory responses may be triggered by various factors, including infections, autoimmune reactions, and environmental toxins.

6. Vascular Factors: Reduced blood flow to the brain, as seen in conditions such as stroke or small vessel disease, can lead to damage in the substantia nigra. Vascular insults can deprive neurons of oxygen and nutrients, leading to cell death and dysfunction.

7. Traumatic Brain Injury: Severe head trauma or repeated concussions can cause damage to various brain regions, including the substantia nigra. Traumatic brain injury can lead to neuronal loss, disruption of neural circuits, and the development of neurodegenerative changes over time.

Substantia nigra and other neuro transmitters

The substantia nigra interacts with other neurotransmitters, including dopamine and GABA (gamma-aminobutyric acid), to regulate various brain functions, particularly those related to movement and motor control.

1. Dopamine:
   - Dopamine is a neurotransmitter that plays a crucial role in modulating movement, motivation, reward, and cognition.
   - The substantia nigra contains dopaminergic neurons in its pars compacta region, which project to the striatum and other brain regions.
   - Dopamine released from the substantia nigra modulates the activity of the basal ganglia, a group of interconnected brain structures involved in motor planning and execution.
   - Dysfunction of dopaminergic neurons in the substantia nigra is associated with movement disorders such as Parkinson's disease, characterized by motor symptoms like tremors, rigidity, and bradykinesia.

2. GABA:

- GABA is the main inhibitory neurotransmitter in the brain, acting to reduce neuronal excitability and regulate neural activity.
- The substantia nigra contains GABAergic neurons in its pars reticulata region, which project to various brain regions including the thalamus, superior colliculus, and brainstem nuclei.
- GABAergic projections from the substantia nigra pars reticulata exert inhibitory control over target structures, contributing to the modulation of motor function, eye movements, and other physiological processes.
- Imbalances in GABAergic neurotransmission within the substantia nigra have been implicated in movement disorders such as Parkinson's disease and dystonia, highlighting the importance of GABAergic signaling in motor control.

In summary, the substantia nigra interacts with neurotransmitters such as dopamine and GABA to regulate motor function and other brain processes. Dysfunction of dopaminergic and GABAergic systems within the substantia nigra can lead to movement disorders and other neurological conditions, underscoring the importance of balanced neurotransmission for healthy brain function.

Treatment??

While there is currently no therapy that can directly repair damage to the substantia nigra, several interventions can help manage symptoms and potentially slow the progression of neurodegenerative diseases like Parkinson's:

1. Physical Therapy and Exercise: Physical therapy and regular exercise are essential components of Parkinson's disease management. Exercise programs tailored to individuals with Parkinson's can help improve mobility, balance, flexibility, and overall physical function. Activities such as walking, cycling, tai chi, yoga, and dance have been shown to be beneficial. Exercise may also have neuroprotective effects and promote neuroplasticity in the brain.

2. Occupational Therapy: Occupational therapy can help individuals with Parkinson's disease maintain independence in activities of daily living. Therapists can provide strategies and adaptations to overcome difficulties with fine motor skills, self-care tasks, and household activities. They may also recommend assistive devices and adaptive equipment to improve functional abilities.

3. Speech and Swallowing Therapy: Parkinson's disease can affect speech and swallowing function due to changes in muscle control and coordination. Speech therapy can help improve speech clarity, volume, and swallowing function through exercises, techniques, and strategies. Therapists may also recommend dietary modifications and swallowing exercises to reduce the risk of aspiration.

4. Cognitive Rehabilitation: Some individuals with Parkinson's disease may experience cognitive changes, such as memory problems, executive dysfunction, and attention deficits. Cognitive rehabilitation programs can target specific cognitive domains through cognitive exercises, memory strategies, and problem-solving tasks. These interventions aim to optimize cognitive function and maintain independence in daily activities.

5. Virtual Reality (VR) Therapy: Virtual reality has emerged as a promising tool for rehabilitation in Parkinson's disease. VR-based interventions can provide immersive and engaging environments for motor training, balance exercises, and gait rehabilitation. Virtual reality systems can simulate real-world activities and challenges while providing feedback and motivation to users.

6. Assistive Devices: Various assistive devices and technologies can help individuals with Parkinson's disease compensate for motor impairments and enhance independence. These devices may include mobility aids (such as walkers or canes), adaptive utensils, voice-activated devices, tremor-reducing orthoses, and specialized computer software.

7. Social and Recreational Activities: Engaging in social and recreational activities can improve mood, reduce stress, and enhance overall well-being for individuals with Parkinson's disease. Participation in hobbies, games, group exercise classes, support groups, and community events can provide social interaction, stimulation, and a sense of belonging.

While these therapies cannot reverse damage to the substantia nigra, they can help manage symptoms, improve quality of life, and promote functional independence for individuals living with Parkinson's disease and other neurodegenerative disorders. It's important for individuals with Parkinson's to work with a multidisciplinary team of healthcare professionals to develop a comprehensive treatment plan tailored to their specific needs and goals.

Role in gambling and addiction

The substantia nigra is indirectly involved in gambling addiction and other addictive behaviors that involve the dopaminergic system. While the substantia nigra itself is not typically the primary locus of dysfunction in these disorders, its connections with other brain regions, particularly those within the mesolimbic dopamine system, play a significant role.

1. Mesolimbic Dopamine System: The mesolimbic dopamine system, which includes dopaminergic neurons originating in the ventral tegmental area (VTA) and projecting to regions such as the nucleus accumbens, amygdala, and prefrontal cortex, is heavily involved in reward processing and reinforcement learning. This system plays a crucial role in mediating the rewarding effects of addictive substances and behaviors.

2. Dopamine Release: During gambling and other rewarding activities, there is an increase in dopamine release in the mesolimbic system, including projections from the VTA to the nucleus accumbens. This dopamine release is associated with feelings of pleasure, motivation, and reinforcement, reinforcing

the behavior and increasing the likelihood of repetition.

3. Role of Substantia Nigra: While the substantia nigra is not directly part of the mesolimbic dopamine system, it is functionally connected to regions involved in reward processing, including the nucleus accumbens. The substantia nigra contributes to the regulation of dopamine release in these regions, indirectly influencing reward-related behaviors.

4. Dysregulation in Addiction: In addiction, including gambling addiction, there is dysregulation of the dopamine system, leading to heightened sensitivity to rewarding stimuli and impaired impulse control. While the exact mechanisms underlying addiction are complex and multifaceted, dysfunction in dopaminergic pathways, including those involving the substantia nigra, is implicated in the development and maintenance of addictive behaviors.

5. Neuroplasticity and Conditioning: Chronic exposure to addictive substances or behaviors can lead to neuroplastic changes in the brain, including alterations in dopamine receptor sensitivity and synaptic connectivity. These changes contribute to the establishment of conditioned responses to cues

associated with the addictive behavior, perpetuating the cycle of addiction.

Thus, while the substantia nigra itself is not the primary site of dysfunction in gambling addiction or other addictive behaviors, its connections with other dopaminergic regions within the brain contribute to the regulation of reward processing and reinforcement learning. Dysregulation of the dopaminergic system, including alterations in dopamine release and receptor sensitivity, is implicated in the development and maintenance of addictive behaviors.

Activation of substantia nigra

The substantia nigra is activated through complex neural circuitry involving various brain regions and neurotransmitter systems. Its activation is primarily modulated by the interplay between excitatory and inhibitory inputs from different brain regions. Here's an overview of how the substantia nigra is activated:

1. Excitatory Inputs: The substantia nigra receives excitatory inputs from several brain regions, including the cortex, thalamus, and limbic system structures such as the amygdala and hippocampus. These excitatory inputs convey information about sensory stimuli, motor commands, and reward-related signals to the substantia nigra.

2. Dopaminergic Inputs: Dopaminergic neurons within the substantia nigra pars compacta (SNc) receive modulatory inputs from dopaminergic neurons originating in the ventral tegmental area (VTA). These dopaminergic projections play a crucial role in regulating the activity of substantia nigra neurons and modulating their responsiveness to excitatory inputs.

3. Inhibitory Inputs: The substantia nigra also receives inhibitory inputs from other basal ganglia

structures, including the striatum (specifically the direct and indirect pathways), globus pallidus, and subthalamic nucleus. These inhibitory inputs help to regulate the output of substantia nigra neurons and modulate their activity in response to incoming signals.

4. Functional Connectivity: The substantia nigra is functionally connected to other brain regions involved in motor control, reward processing, and cognitive function, such as the striatum, globus pallidus, thalamus, and cortex. These connections form intricate neural circuits that regulate motor behavior, decision-making, and reinforcement learning.

5. Activation by Salient Stimuli: The substantia nigra can be activated by salient stimuli, including rewarding or aversive cues, novel experiences, and motor commands. Activation of dopaminergic neurons in the substantia nigra is associated with the processing of reward prediction errors, which play a crucial role in reinforcement learning and decision-making.

6. Role in Movement Initiation: Activation of the substantia nigra is essential for initiating and modulating voluntary movements. Dopaminergic

neurons in the substantia nigra pars compacta (SNc) project to the striatum and other basal ganglia nuclei, where they regulate the initiation and execution of motor commands.

Role of caffeine in substantia nigra

Caffeine, a well-known psychoactive substance found in coffee, tea, and various other beverages and foods, can affect the substantia nigra and dopaminergic activity through its actions on adenosine receptors.

1. Adenosine Receptor Antagonism: Caffeine exerts its effects by antagonizing adenosine receptors in the brain. Adenosine is a neurotransmitter that acts as an endogenous neuromodulator and has inhibitory effects on neuronal activity. By blocking adenosine receptors, caffeine increases neuronal excitability and neurotransmitter release, including dopamine.

2. Effect on Dopaminergic Neurons: The substantia nigra contains dopaminergic neurons that are critical for motor control and reward processing. Caffeine's blockade of adenosine receptors, particularly the A2A subtype, leads to increased firing rates of dopaminergic neurons in the substantia nigra and other regions of the brain.

3. Enhancement of Dopamine Release: By promoting the activity of dopaminergic neurons in the substantia nigra, caffeine can enhance dopamine release in target areas such as the striatum and prefrontal cortex. This increase in dopamine

transmission contributes to caffeine's stimulant effects and may influence mood, attention, and motor function.

4. Potential Therapeutic Effects: Research suggests that caffeine's modulation of dopaminergic activity in the substantia nigra and other brain regions may have therapeutic implications for neurological and neuropsychiatric disorders. For example, caffeine has been investigated for its potential neuroprotective effects in Parkinson's disease, as it may help mitigate dopaminergic neuron loss and motor symptoms.

5. Behavioral Effects: The activation of dopaminergic pathways by caffeine can also influence behavior. Caffeine consumption is associated with increased alertness, arousal, and locomotor activity, which are mediated in part by its effects on the substantia nigra and other dopaminergic brain regions.

In relation to Parkinson's disease…

The substantia nigra plays a crucial role in both the treatment and research of Parkinson's disease due to its central involvement in the pathophysiology of the disorder:

1. Treatment:
   - Medication Targets: Many medications used to manage Parkinson's disease target the dopaminergic system, which is primarily affected by the degeneration of neurons in the substantia nigra. These medications aim to increase dopamine levels in the brain, alleviate motor symptoms, and improve overall quality of life for individuals with Parkinson's.
   - Deep Brain Stimulation (DBS): Deep brain stimulation, a surgical procedure that involves implanting electrodes into specific brain regions, including the substantia nigra, is an effective treatment option for individuals with advanced Parkinson's disease. DBS can help alleviate motor symptoms such as tremors, rigidity, and bradykinesia by modulating neural activity in the substantia nigra and other basal ganglia structures.
   - Neuroprotection Research: Given the central role of the substantia nigra in Parkinson's disease pathology, research efforts are focused on developing neuroprotective therapies that can slow or halt the

progression of the disease. Targeting mechanisms involved in neuronal degeneration and dysfunction in the substantia nigra is a key area of investigation for potential disease-modifying treatments.

2. Research:

- Pathophysiology Studies: Research into the pathophysiology of Parkinson's disease often involves studying the cellular and molecular changes that occur in the substantia nigra and other brain regions affected by the disease. Understanding the underlying mechanisms of neuronal degeneration and dysfunction in the substantia nigra is essential for developing targeted therapies and interventions.

- Biomarker Development: Identifying reliable biomarkers associated with substantia nigra dysfunction could aid in the early diagnosis and monitoring of Parkinson's disease progression. Biomarker research may involve imaging techniques such as MRI and PET scans to detect changes in substantia nigra structure and function.

- Novel Therapeutic Targets: Investigating novel therapeutic targets within the substantia nigra and its neural circuits holds promise for developing more effective treatments for Parkinson's disease. Research efforts may focus on neurotrophic factors, gene therapy, stem cell-based therapies, and other innovative approaches to restore dopaminergic function and protect neurons in the substantia nigra.

Substantia nigra in other animals

The substantia nigra is a brain structure found not only in humans but also in other vertebrate animals, including mammals, birds, and reptiles. While there may be variations in size, organization, and function across species, the general anatomical and functional characteristics of the substantia nigra are conserved. Here's how the substantia nigra appears in other animals:

1. Mammals:
   - In mammals, the substantia nigra consists of two main regions: the pars compacta (SNc) and the pars reticulata (SNr).
   - The SNc contains dopaminergic neurons that project to the striatum and are involved in motor control and reward processing.
   - The SNr contains GABAergic neurons that project to various brain regions and are involved in modulating movement, attention, and other functions.

2. Birds:
   - Birds also possess a substantia nigra with similar anatomical features to mammals, including dopaminergic and GABAergic neurons.

- Studies in birds have demonstrated the involvement of the substantia nigra in motor control, vocalization, and other behaviors.

3. Reptiles:
   - Reptiles such as reptiles have a less developed substantia nigra compared to mammals and birds, but they still possess dopaminergic and GABAergic neurons within this brain region.
   - The substantia nigra in reptiles is involved in regulating motor behavior, thermoregulation, and other physiological functions.

While the specific functions and neural circuits involving the substantia nigra may vary across species, its fundamental role in motor control and other brain processes appears to be evolutionarily conserved. Studying the substantia nigra in different animal models provides valuable insights into its function and dysfunction across diverse biological contexts, contributing to our understanding of brain evolution and neurological disorders.

Summary

Let's break down the substantia nigra in terms of its anatomy, functions, usage, and strategies for maintaining and improving its functions:

1. Anatomy:
    - The substantia nigra is a small, ovoid structure located in the midbrain, specifically within the mesencephalon.
    - It is divided into two main parts: the substantia nigra pars compacta (SNc) and the substantia nigra pars reticulata (SNr).
    - The SNc contains dopamine-producing neurons that project to the striatum and are involved in motor control.
    - The SNr contains GABAergic neurons that project to various brain regions and are involved in modulating movement, as well as other functions such as attention and reward processing.

2. Functions:
    - The substantia nigra plays a critical role in the regulation of movement, particularly through its dopaminergic projections to the striatum.
    - Dopamine released from the substantia nigra helps modulate the activity of the basal ganglia, a

group of structures involved in motor planning and execution.

- Dysfunction of the substantia nigra, such as the loss of dopaminergic neurons seen in Parkinson's disease, can lead to motor symptoms such as tremors, rigidity, and bradykinesia.

3. Usage:

- The substantia nigra is actively engaged during voluntary movements, including both gross motor activities (e.g., walking, reaching) and fine motor tasks (e.g., writing, buttoning a shirt).
- It is also involved in various cognitive functions, including attention, executive function, and reward processing.
- Dysfunction of the substantia nigra can impact not only movement but also cognitive and emotional processes.

4. Maintaining and Improving Functions:

- Physical Exercise: Regular physical activity, including aerobic exercise, strength training, and activities that challenge balance and coordination, can help maintain and improve substantia nigra function.
- Healthy Lifestyle: Adopting a healthy lifestyle that includes a balanced diet, adequate sleep, stress management, and avoidance of harmful substances

(e.g., excessive alcohol, smoking) can support overall brain health, including the substantia nigra.

- Brain Training: Engaging in activities that stimulate cognitive function, such as puzzles, games, learning new skills, and social interactions, can help maintain cognitive abilities associated with the substantia nigra.

- Medication and Therapy: For individuals with Parkinson's disease or other neurological disorders affecting the substantia nigra, medications, deep brain stimulation, physical therapy, occupational therapy, and speech therapy can help manage symptoms and improve quality of life.

In summary, the substantia nigra is a vital brain structure involved in movement, cognition, and emotion. Maintaining its function requires a combination of lifestyle factors, physical activity, cognitive stimulation, and appropriate medical interventions for individuals with neurological conditions affecting the substantia nigra.

www.ingramcontent.com/pod-product-compliance
Lightning Source LLC
Chambersburg PA
CBHW031556210526
45464CB00003B/1315